MW00378451

THIS *planner* BELONGS TO:

Patti Claire Denman

meal planner

MONDAY	
TUESDAY	
WEDNESDAY	
THURSDAY	
FRIDAY	
SATURDAY	
SUNDAY	

WEEK OF: *Monday* ______________, 20__

grocery list

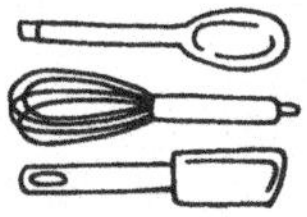

meal planner

MONDAY	
TUESDAY	
WEDNESDAY	
THURSDAY	
FRIDAY	
SATURDAY	
SUNDAY	

WEEK OF: Monday ____________________, 20__

grocery list

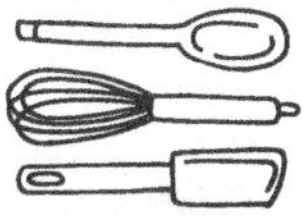

meal planner

MONDAY	
TUESDAY	
WEDNESDAY	
THURSDAY	
FRIDAY	
SATURDAY	
SUNDAY	

WEEK OF: *Monday* ______________, 20__

grocery list

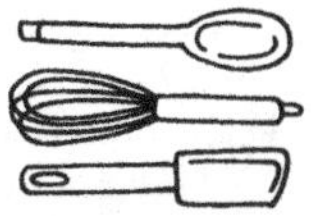

meal planner

MONDAY	
TUESDAY	
WEDNESDAY	
THURSDAY	
FRIDAY	
SATURDAY	
SUNDAY	

WEEK OF: *Monday* ______________, 20__

grocery list

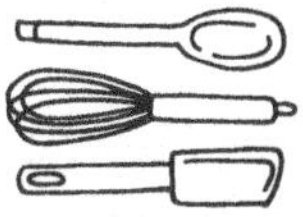

meal planner

MONDAY	
TUESDAY	
WEDNESDAY	
THURSDAY	
FRIDAY	
SATURDAY	
SUNDAY	

WEEK OF: *Monday* ____________, 20__

grocery list

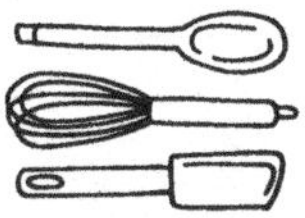

meal planner

MONDAY	
TUESDAY	
WEDNESDAY	
THURSDAY	
FRIDAY	
SATURDAY	
SUNDAY	

WEEK OF: *Monday* ____________, 20__

grocery list

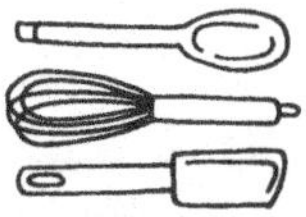

meal planner

MONDAY	
TUESDAY	
WEDNESDAY	
THURSDAY	
FRIDAY	
SATURDAY	
SUNDAY	

WEEK OF: Monday ________________, 20__

grocery list

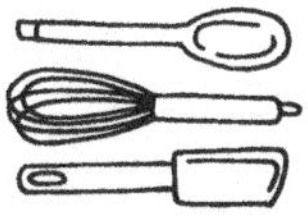

meal planner

MONDAY	
TUESDAY	
WEDNESDAY	
THURSDAY	
FRIDAY	
SATURDAY	
SUNDAY	

WEEK OF: *Monday* ________________, 20__

grocery list

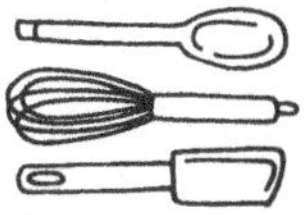

meal planner

MONDAY	
TUESDAY	
WEDNESDAY	
THURSDAY	
FRIDAY	
SATURDAY	
SUNDAY	

WEEK OF: *Monday* ____________, 20__

grocery list

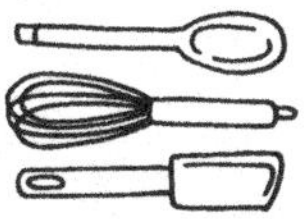

meal planner

MONDAY	
TUESDAY	
WEDNESDAY	
THURSDAY	
FRIDAY	
SATURDAY	
SUNDAY	

WEEK OF: *Monday* ______________, 20__

grocery list

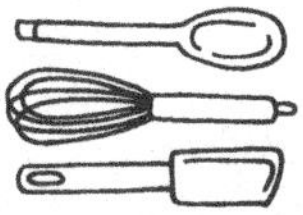

meal planner

MONDAY	
TUESDAY	
WEDNESDAY	
THURSDAY	
FRIDAY	
SATURDAY	
SUNDAY	

WEEK OF: *Monday* ______________, 20__

grocery list

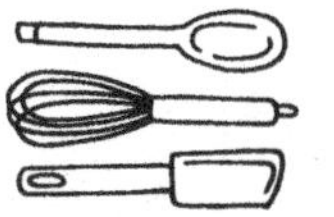

meal planner

MONDAY	
TUESDAY	
WEDNESDAY	
THURSDAY	
FRIDAY	
SATURDAY	
SUNDAY	

WEEK OF: Monday ________________, 20__

grocery list

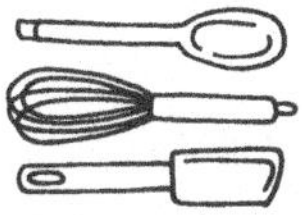

meal planner

MONDAY	
TUESDAY	
WEDNESDAY	
THURSDAY	
FRIDAY	
SATURDAY	
SUNDAY	

WEEK OF: *Monday* ______________, 20__

grocery list

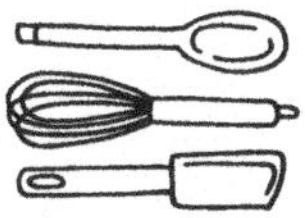

meal planner

MONDAY	
TUESDAY	
WEDNESDAY	
THURSDAY	
FRIDAY	
SATURDAY	
SUNDAY	

WEEK OF: *Monday* ______________, 20__

grocery list

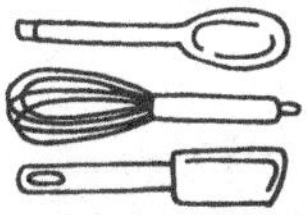

meal planner

MONDAY	
TUESDAY	
WEDNESDAY	
THURSDAY	
FRIDAY	
SATURDAY	
SUNDAY	

WEEK OF: *Monday* ____________, 20__

grocery list

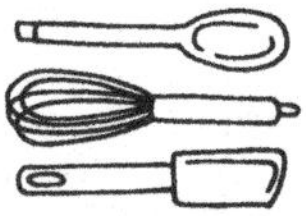

meal planner

MONDAY	
TUESDAY	
WEDNESDAY	
THURSDAY	
FRIDAY	
SATURDAY	
SUNDAY	

WEEK OF: *Monday* ________________, 20__

grocery list

- [ ] ______________________________
- [ ] ______________________________
- [ ] ______________________________
- [ ] ______________________________
- [ ] ______________________________
- [ ] ______________________________
- [ ] ______________________________
- [ ] ______________________________
- [ ] ______________________________
- [ ] ______________________________
- [ ] ______________________________
- [ ] ______________________________
- [ ] ______________________________
- [ ] ______________________________
- [ ] ______________________________
- [ ] ______________________________
- [ ] ______________________________
- [ ] ______________________________
- [ ] ______________________________
- [ ] ______________________________
- [ ] ______________________________
- [ ] ______________________________
- [ ] ______________________________
- [ ] ______________________________
- [ ] ______________________________
- [ ] ______________________________
- [ ] ______________________________
- [ ] ______________________________
- [ ] ______________________________
- [ ] ______________________________
- [ ] ______________________________
- [ ] ______________________________
- [ ] ______________________________
- [ ] ______________________________
- [ ] ______________________________
- [ ] ______________________________
- [ ] ______________________________
- [ ] ______________________________
- [ ] ______________________________
- [ ] ______________________________
- [ ] ______________________________
- [ ] ______________________________
- [ ] ______________________________
- [ ] ______________________________
- [ ] ______________________________
- [ ] ______________________________
- [ ] ______________________________
- [ ] ______________________________
- [ ] ______________________________
- [ ] ______________________________
- [ ] ______________________________
- [ ] ______________________________

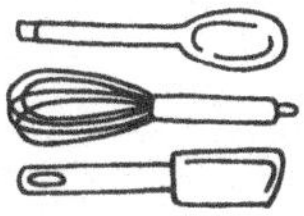

meal planner

MONDAY	
TUESDAY	
WEDNESDAY	
THURSDAY	
FRIDAY	
SATURDAY	
SUNDAY	

WEEK OF: *Monday* ____________________, 20__

grocery list

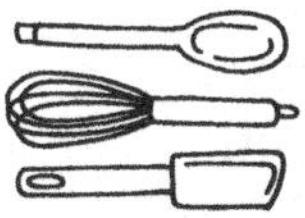

meal planner

MONDAY	
TUESDAY	
WEDNESDAY	
THURSDAY	
FRIDAY	
SATURDAY	
SUNDAY	

WEEK OF: *Monday* ________________, 20__

grocery list

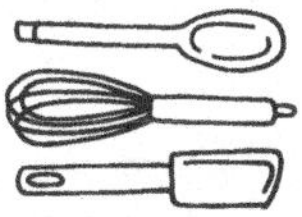

meal planner

MONDAY	
TUESDAY	
WEDNESDAY	
THURSDAY	
FRIDAY	
SATURDAY	
SUNDAY	

WEEK OF: *Monday* ______________, 20__

grocery list

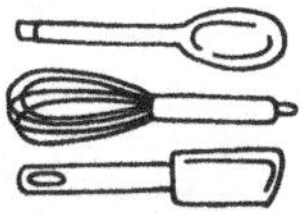

meal planner

MONDAY	
TUESDAY	
WEDNESDAY	
THURSDAY	
FRIDAY	
SATURDAY	
SUNDAY	

WEEK OF: Monday __________________, 20__

grocery list

meal planner

MONDAY	
TUESDAY	
WEDNESDAY	
THURSDAY	
FRIDAY	
SATURDAY	
SUNDAY	

WEEK OF: *Monday* ______________, 20__

grocery list

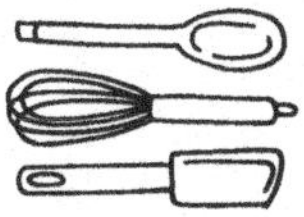

meal planner

MONDAY	
TUESDAY	
WEDNESDAY	
THURSDAY	
FRIDAY	
SATURDAY	
SUNDAY	

WEEK OF: *Monday* ________________, 20__

grocery list

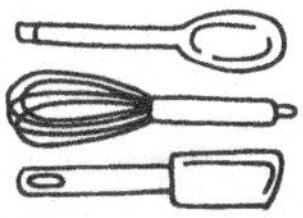

meal planner

MONDAY	
TUESDAY	
WEDNESDAY	
THURSDAY	
FRIDAY	
SATURDAY	
SUNDAY	

WEEK OF: *Monday* ____________________, 20__

grocery list

- [ ]
- [ ]
- [ ]
- [ ]
- [ ]
- [ ]
- [ ]
- [ ]
- [ ]
- [ ]
- [ ]
- [ ]
- [ ]
- [ ]
- [ ]
- [ ]
- [ ]
- [ ]
- [ ]
- [ ]
- [ ]
- [ ]
- [ ]
- [ ]
- [ ]
- [ ]

- [ ]
- [ ]
- [ ]
- [ ]
- [ ]
- [ ]
- [ ]
- [ ]
- [ ]
- [ ]
- [ ]
- [ ]
- [ ]
- [ ]
- [ ]
- [ ]
- [ ]
- [ ]
- [ ]
- [ ]
- [ ]
- [ ]
- [ ]
- [ ]
- [ ]
- [ ]

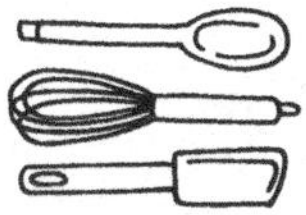

meal planner

MONDAY	
TUESDAY	
WEDNESDAY	
THURSDAY	
FRIDAY	
SATURDAY	
SUNDAY	

WEEK OF: *Monday* ________________, 20__

grocery list

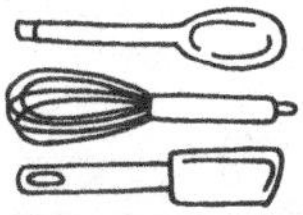

meal planner

MONDAY	
TUESDAY	
WEDNESDAY	
THURSDAY	
FRIDAY	
SATURDAY	
SUNDAY	

WEEK OF: *Monday* ______________, 20__

grocery list

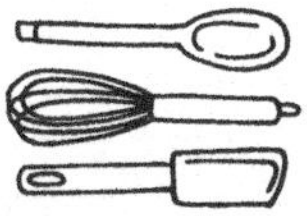

meal planner

MONDAY	
TUESDAY	
WEDNESDAY	
THURSDAY	
FRIDAY	
SATURDAY	
SUNDAY	

WEEK OF: *Monday* ____________, 20__

grocery list

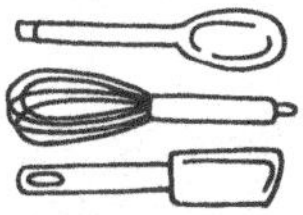

meal planner

MONDAY	
TUESDAY	
WEDNESDAY	
THURSDAY	
FRIDAY	
SATURDAY	
SUNDAY	

WEEK OF: *Monday* ____________________, 20__

grocery list

- [ ]
- [ ]
- [ ]
- [ ]
- [ ]
- [ ]
- [ ]
- [ ]
- [ ]
- [ ]
- [ ]
- [ ]
- [ ]
- [ ]
- [ ]
- [ ]
- [ ]
- [ ]
- [ ]
- [ ]
- [ ]
- [ ]
- [ ]
- [ ]
- [ ]
- [ ]
- [ ]
- [ ]
- [ ]
- [ ]
- [ ]
- [ ]
- [ ]
- [ ]
- [ ]
- [ ]
- [ ]
- [ ]
- [ ]
- [ ]
- [ ]
- [ ]
- [ ]
- [ ]
- [ ]
- [ ]
- [ ]
- [ ]
- [ ]
- [ ]
- [ ]
- [ ]

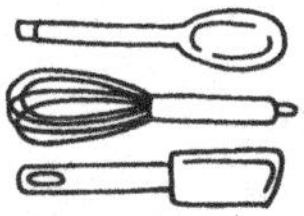

meal planner

MONDAY	
TUESDAY	
WEDNESDAY	
THURSDAY	
FRIDAY	
SATURDAY	
SUNDAY	

WEEK OF: *Monday* ________________, 20__

grocery list

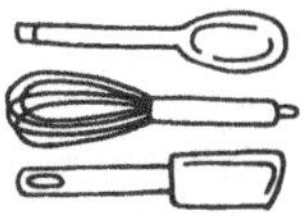

meal planner

MONDAY	
TUESDAY	
WEDNESDAY	
THURSDAY	
FRIDAY	
SATURDAY	
SUNDAY	

WEEK OF: *Monday* ______________, 20__

grocery list

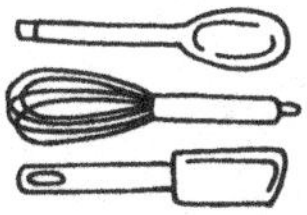

meal planner

MONDAY	
TUESDAY	
WEDNESDAY	
THURSDAY	
FRIDAY	
SATURDAY	
SUNDAY	

WEEK OF: *Monday* _______________, 20__

grocery list

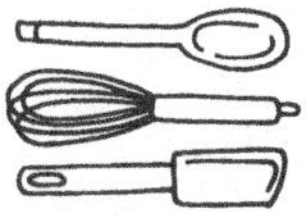

meal planner

MONDAY	
TUESDAY	
WEDNESDAY	
THURSDAY	
FRIDAY	
SATURDAY	
SUNDAY	

WEEK OF: *Monday* ______________, 20__

grocery list

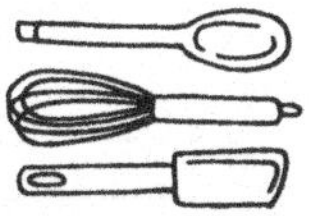

meal planner

MONDAY	
TUESDAY	
WEDNESDAY	
THURSDAY	
FRIDAY	
SATURDAY	
SUNDAY	

WEEK OF: *Monday* ____________________, 20__

grocery list

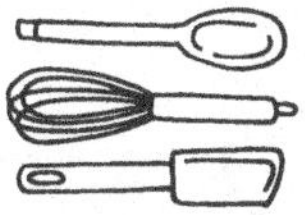

meal planner

MONDAY	
TUESDAY	
WEDNESDAY	
THURSDAY	
FRIDAY	
SATURDAY	
SUNDAY	

WEEK OF: *Monday* ______________, 20__

grocery list

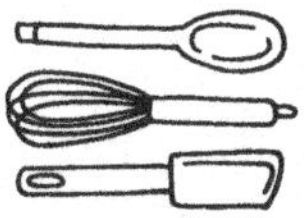

meal planner

MONDAY	
TUESDAY	
WEDNESDAY	
THURSDAY	
FRIDAY	
SATURDAY	
SUNDAY	

WEEK OF: *Monday* ____________________, 20__

grocery list

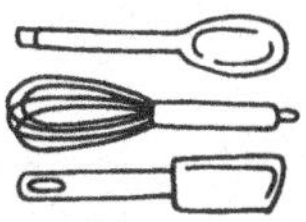

meal planner

MONDAY	
TUESDAY	
WEDNESDAY	
THURSDAY	
FRIDAY	
SATURDAY	
SUNDAY	

WEEK OF: *Monday* ______________, 20__

grocery list

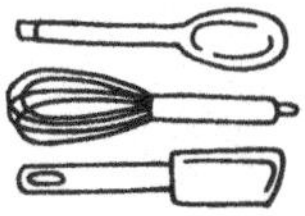

meal planner

MONDAY	
TUESDAY	
WEDNESDAY	
THURSDAY	
FRIDAY	
SATURDAY	
SUNDAY	

WEEK OF: *Monday* ____________, 20__

grocery list

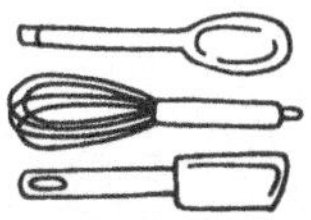

meal planner

MONDAY	
TUESDAY	
WEDNESDAY	
THURSDAY	
FRIDAY	
SATURDAY	
SUNDAY	

WEEK OF: *Monday* ______________, 20__

grocery list

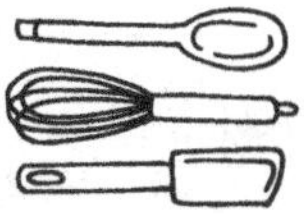

meal planner

MONDAY	
TUESDAY	
WEDNESDAY	
THURSDAY	
FRIDAY	
SATURDAY	
SUNDAY	

WEEK OF: *Monday* ________________, 20__

grocery list

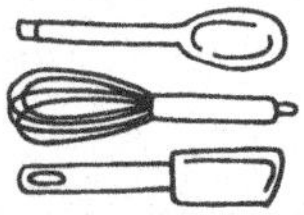

meal planner

MONDAY	
TUESDAY	
WEDNESDAY	
THURSDAY	
FRIDAY	
SATURDAY	
SUNDAY	

WEEK OF: *Monday* ______________, 20__

grocery list

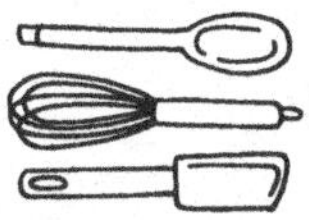

meal planner

MONDAY	
TUESDAY	
WEDNESDAY	
THURSDAY	
FRIDAY	
SATURDAY	
SUNDAY	

WEEK OF: *Monday* ________________, 20__

grocery list

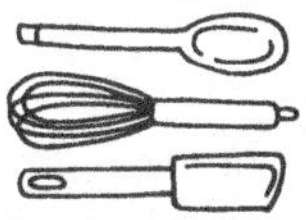

meal planner

MONDAY	
TUESDAY	
WEDNESDAY	
THURSDAY	
FRIDAY	
SATURDAY	
SUNDAY	

WEEK OF: *Monday* ________________, 20__

grocery list

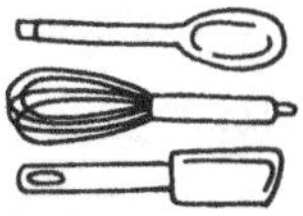

meal planner

MONDAY	
TUESDAY	
WEDNESDAY	
THURSDAY	
FRIDAY	
SATURDAY	
SUNDAY	

WEEK OF: *Monday* ______________, 20__

grocery list

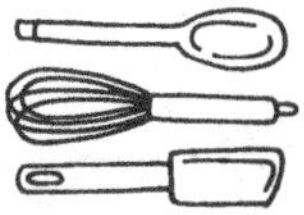

meal planner

MONDAY	
TUESDAY	
WEDNESDAY	
THURSDAY	
FRIDAY	
SATURDAY	
SUNDAY	

WEEK OF: Monday ________________, 20__

grocery list

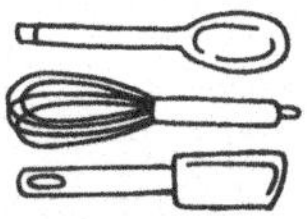

meal planner

MONDAY	
TUESDAY	
WEDNESDAY	
THURSDAY	
FRIDAY	
SATURDAY	
SUNDAY	

WEEK OF: *Monday* __________________, 20__

grocery list

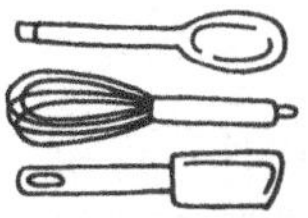

meal planner

MONDAY	
TUESDAY	
WEDNESDAY	
THURSDAY	
FRIDAY	
SATURDAY	
SUNDAY	

WEEK OF: *Monday* __________________, 20__

grocery list

- [ ]
- [ ]
- [ ]
- [ ]
- [ ]
- [ ]
- [ ]
- [ ]
- [ ]
- [ ]
- [ ]
- [ ]
- [ ]
- [ ]
- [ ]
- [ ]
- [ ]
- [ ]
- [ ]
- [ ]
- [ ]
- [ ]
- [ ]
- [ ]
- [ ]
- [ ]
- [ ]
- [ ]
- [ ]
- [ ]
- [ ]
- [ ]
- [ ]
- [ ]
- [ ]
- [ ]
- [ ]
- [ ]
- [ ]
- [ ]
- [ ]
- [ ]
- [ ]
- [ ]
- [ ]
- [ ]
- [ ]
- [ ]
- [ ]
- [ ]
- [ ]
- [ ]

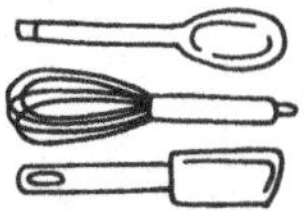

meal planner

MONDAY	
TUESDAY	
WEDNESDAY	
THURSDAY	
FRIDAY	
SATURDAY	
SUNDAY	

WEEK OF: *Monday* ______________________, 20__

grocery list

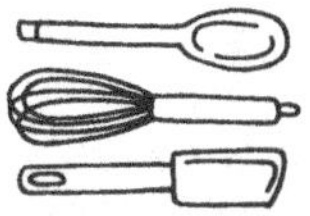

meal planner

MONDAY	
TUESDAY	
WEDNESDAY	
THURSDAY	
FRIDAY	
SATURDAY	
SUNDAY	

WEEK OF: Monday ______________, 20__

grocery list

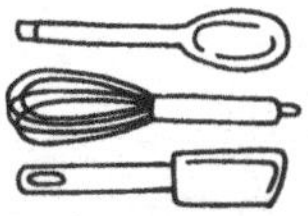

meal planner

MONDAY	
TUESDAY	
WEDNESDAY	
THURSDAY	
FRIDAY	
SATURDAY	
SUNDAY	

WEEK OF: Monday ______________, 20__

grocery list

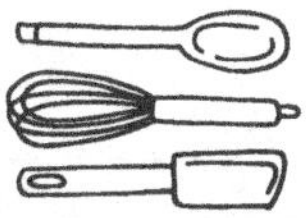

meal planner

MONDAY	
TUESDAY	
WEDNESDAY	
THURSDAY	
FRIDAY	
SATURDAY	
SUNDAY	

WEEK OF: *Monday* ______________________, 20__

grocery list

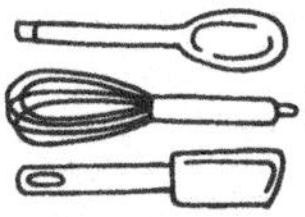

meal planner

MONDAY	
TUESDAY	
WEDNESDAY	
THURSDAY	
FRIDAY	
SATURDAY	
SUNDAY	

WEEK OF: *Monday* ____________________, 20__

grocery list

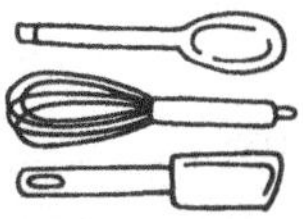

meal planner

MONDAY	
TUESDAY	
WEDNESDAY	
THURSDAY	
FRIDAY	
SATURDAY	
SUNDAY	

WEEK OF: *Monday* ______________, 20__

grocery list

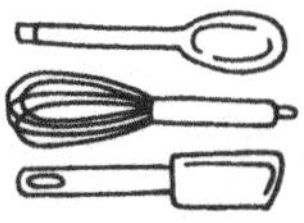

meal planner

MONDAY	
TUESDAY	
WEDNESDAY	
THURSDAY	
FRIDAY	
SATURDAY	
SUNDAY	

WEEK OF: *Monday* ____________, 20__

grocery list

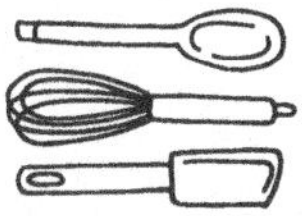

meal planner

MONDAY	
TUESDAY	
WEDNESDAY	
THURSDAY	
FRIDAY	
SATURDAY	
SUNDAY	

WEEK OF: *Monday* ____________________, 20__

grocery list

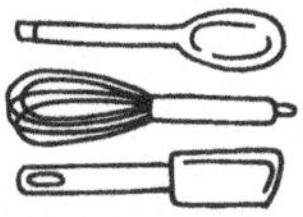

Made in the USA
Las Vegas, NV
12 October 2023

78998972R00063